HOW TO GET PREGNANT

FOOD TO MAKE A WOMAN PREGNANT IMMEDIATELY

ALEXIS SARRATT

TABLE OF CONTENT

Introduction

Many people believe that getting pregnant is a simple, natural procedure. However, a woman's capacity to conceive can be impacted by a variety of variables, including age, weight, and general health. Nutrition is a critical factor that is sometimes disregarded.

Our diet has a big impact on how healthy we are reproductively, affecting everything from hormone balance to the quality of our eggs.

According to studies, women who eat a balanced, healthy diet are more likely to conceive and deliver healthy babies. Contrarily, those who consume a diet heavy in processed foods and sugar are more likely to experience infertility problems and issues during pregnancy.

It is impossible to exaggerate the significance of nutrition for fertility. Healthy fats and proteins are critical for hormone balance and overall reproductive health, while nutrients like folate, iron, and calcium are crucial for fetal development.

Women can increase their chances of getting pregnant and having a healthy pregnancy by emphasizing a diet high in certain nutrients.

It can be difficult to decide which meals to eat and which to avoid. "How to Get Pregnant: Food to Make a Woman Pregnant Immediately" can be a helpful tool in this situation.

This book offers a thorough overview of using nutrition to increase conception and lists the precise foods and nutrients that are most helpful for women who are attempting to get pregnant.

The principles of fertility and the function of nutrition in conception, important nutrients for fertility, foods for better egg quality and hormone management, and dietary suggestions for optimal fertility are just a few of the topics covered in the book.

Additionally, it answers frequent queries and worries about nutrition and conception, such as whether or not it is safe to consume caffeine while pregnant and how much protein is required for optimum fertility.

Women can boost their chances of getting pregnant and improve their general health by following the advice provided in the book.

Consuming a diet high in whole, nutrient-dense foods, avoiding processed and sugary meals, drinking enough water, and taking supplements with important nutrients when needed are all part of this.

The book offers helpful advice for enhancing general reproductive health in addition to dietary recommendations.

This entails preserving a healthy weight, engaging in regular exercise, controlling stress, and avoiding pollutants that may harm fertility.

In the end, "How to Get Pregnant: Food to Make a Woman Pregnant Immediately" is a priceless tool for any woman attempting to get pregnant.

Women can increase their chances of getting pregnant and having a healthy pregnancy by recognizing the crucial role that nutrition plays in fertility and making appropriate dietary and lifestyle modifications.

This book offers insightful information and helpful suggestions that can aid in your quest to conceive, regardless of how far along you are in your fertility journey or how long you have been trying.

Chapter 1

Understanding Fertility

Anyone who is attempting to get pregnant has to understand the fundamentals of fertility because it is a complicated subject. The menstrual cycle, ovulation, potential influences on fertility, and the function of nutrition in fertility are all topics covered in this chapter.

The cycle of Menstruation and Ovulation

Each month, a woman's body gets ready for pregnancy through the menstrual cycle. A complicated interaction of hormones, including progesterone and estrogen, controls it. Although it might vary from woman to woman, the menstrual cycle normally lasts 28 days.

Menstrual hemorrhage begins on the first day of the menstrual cycle. The menstrual period lasts from three to seven days and is referred to as such. The follicular phase then starts.

Follicle-stimulating hormone (FSH), which stimulates the formation of follicles in the ovaries, is produced during this phase as the body gets ready for ovulation. One egg is present in each follicle, but only one will develop and be released at ovulation.

On average, ovulation happens on day 14 of the menstrual cycle. At this point, the developed egg is released from the ovary and moves via the fallopian tube to the place where sperm can fertilize it.

If fertilization fails, the egg will disintegrate and the uterine lining will shed during the subsequent menstrual period.

Issues that may Affect Fertility

The fertility of a woman can be affected by a variety of variables. A few of these are:

- **Age:** Women's fertility decreases with age, especially after the age of 35.

- **Weight:** By messing with the hormone balance, being underweight or overweight might affect fertility.

- **Medical problems:** endometriosis and polycystic ovarian syndrome (PCOS) are two disorders that might affect fertility.

- **Smoking:** binge drinking and stress are all examples of lifestyle issues that might affect fertility.

- **Medication:** some pharmaceuticals like chemotherapy agents might affect fertility.

Nutrition's Effect on Fertility

Infertility is greatly influenced by nutrition, which has an impact on everything from hormone regulation to egg quality. The following nutrients are particularly crucial for reproductive health:

- **Folate:** can lower the risk of neural tube abnormalities and is necessary for healthy embryonic development. Leafy greens, legumes, and fortified cereals all contain it.

- **Iron:** An iron deficit might affect fertility since iron is necessary for normal blood flow. Red meat, leafy vegetables, and fortified cereals all contain it.

- **Calcium:** A shortage might affect fertility and is necessary for the development of healthy bones. Leafy greens, dairy products, and drinks with added vitamins all include it.

- **Healthy fats:** They're essential for hormone balance and overall reproductive health and can be found in foods like nuts, seeds, and fatty fish.

Women can increase their chances of getting pregnant and having a healthy baby by focusing on eating a diet high in essential nutrients and avoiding processed and sugary foods.

Anyone wanting to get pregnant must have a basic understanding of fertility. A precise hormonal balance controls the intricate processes of the menstrual cycle and ovulation.

Age, weight, illnesses, and lifestyle choices are just a few of the many variables that might affect fertility.

Certain nutrients, including folate, iron, and calcium, are crucial for reproductive health and have a significant influence on fertility.

Women can increase their chances of getting pregnant and having a healthy pregnancy by being aware of these factors and adapting their food and lifestyle accordingly.

Chapter 2

Key Nutrients for Fertility

A balanced diet is essential for maintaining reproductive health, as was covered in Chapter 1 of this book. We will go more into the individual nutrients—including protein, carbs, fats, vitamins, and minerals—that are crucial for fertility in this chapter.

Protein

A vital component of the body, protein is also important for reproductive health. The growth and repair of tissues, including reproductive cells, depend on amino acids, which are the building blocks of protein. Additionally, amino acids aid in the regulation of hormone synthesis and metabolism, both of which are essential for fertility.

Legumes, nuts, lean meats, fish, poultry, eggs and seeds are all excellent sources of protein. At least 46 grams of protein per day should be consumed by women who are attempting to get pregnant.

Carbohydrates

The body uses carbohydrates as a major source of energy, and they are essential for reproductive health.

Carbohydrates are crucial for women who are attempting to get pregnant because low-carb diets have been related to decreased fertility.

Whole grains, fruits, vegetables, legumes, and whole grains are all excellent sources of carbs. At least 130 grams of carbs should be consumed each day by women who are attempting to get pregnant.

Fats

The regulation of hormones and general reproductive health depend on healthy lipids. Particularly crucial for the growth of the embryonic nervous system and brain are omega-3 fatty acids.

Butter pearls, nuts, seeds, and fatty fish are good sources of healthful fats.

The fact that not all fats are created equally must be noted. Consuming processed and fried foods that are high in saturated and trans fats might harm fertility and should be done in moderation.

Vitamins

Vitamins are necessary nutrients that are extremely important for reproductive health. The following vitamins are some of the most crucial for fertility:

- **Vitamin D:** Vitamin D is crucial for the control of hormones and may affect fertility. Light from the sun, fatty fish, and fortified dairy products are all excellent sources of vitamin D.

- **Vitamin E:** Vitamin E is essential for the health of sperm and eggs. Plant-based foods such as nuts, seeds, and leafy greens are excellent sources of vitamin E.

- **Vitamin C:** Vitamin C plays a role in the control of hormones and may affect fertility. Bell peppers, berries, and citrus fruits are excellent sources of vitamin C.

- **Vitamin B:** The incidence of neural tube abnormalities can be decreased by taking B vitamins, such as folate and B12, which are crucial for good embryonic development. Leafy greens, lentils, and grains that have been fortified are excellent sources of B vitamins.

Minerals

Minerals are necessary minerals that are extremely important for reproductive health. The following minerals are some of the most crucial for fertility:

- **Iron:** Iron is necessary for normal blood flow and may affect fertility. Red meat, leafy greens, and fortified cereals are all excellent sources of iron.

- **Zinc:** Zinc is necessary for the health of sperm and eggs. Oysters, meat, and fortified grains are all excellent sources of zinc.

- **Calcium:** Calcium is important for the growth of strong bones and affects fertility. Dairy products, leafy greens, and liquids with added calcium are all excellent sources of this mineral.

Women can increase their chances of getting pregnant and having a healthy baby by focusing on eating a diet high in certain essential nutrients.

Prenatal vitamins, which are specially prepared to offer the nutrients that are essential for fetal growth, may be helpful for women who are attempting to get pregnant in addition to a balanced diet.

Protein, carbs, good fats, vitamins, and minerals are the specific foods that are particularly crucial for fertility.

The odds of conception can be increased and reproductive health can be enhanced by eating a balanced diet rich in certain nutrients.

Aim to consume at least 130 grams of carbohydrates and 46 grams of protein for women who are trying to get pregnant.

Chapter 3

Foods for Better Egg Quality

We covered the essential nutrients that are crucial for fertility in the previous chapter. This chapter will concentrate on particular meals that can assist in enhancing egg quality, a crucial element in conception and pregnancy.

The health and viability of a woman's eggs are referred to as "egg quality." As women get older, the quality of their eggs may deteriorate, which may make it harder to get pregnant and raise the risk of difficulties. Certain foods can, however, aid in enhancing egg quality and maintaining reproductive health.

Grassy Leaves

The folate found in leafy greens like spinach, kale, and arugula is a crucial B vitamin for reproductive health.

A deficit in the nutrient folate, which is essential for fetal development, can raise the risk of neural tube abnormalities.

In addition to being high in folate, leafy greens are also a good source of antioxidants, which can help improve the quality and prevent damage to the eggs.

A range of fruits and vegetables, nuts, seeds, and whole grains all contain antioxidants, which are vital for good health.

Berries

Antioxidant-rich berries like blueberries, raspberries, and strawberries can help enhance the quality of eggs.

Berries are a strong source of vitamin C, which is crucial for hormone regulation and may affect fertility in addition to its antioxidant characteristics.

According to research, women who consume more berries than those who do not have a higher chance of getting pregnant.

Large Fish

The omega-3 fatty acids found in fatty fish like salmon, mackerel, and sardines are crucial for reproductive health.

Omega-3 fatty acids can improve egg quality, control hormone production, and lower inflammation in the body.

Omega-3 fatty acids are also present in nuts, seeds, and dietary supplements made from algae, in addition to fatty fish.

Eggs

As we discussed in Chapter 2, eggs are a strong source of protein, which is crucial for reproductive health. Eggs are a good source of both protein and choline, which is crucial for the growth of the fetal brain.

According to research, women who eat more eggs have a better chance of getting pregnant than those who eat fewer eggs.

Whole grains

Whole grains are a rich source of complex carbohydrates, which are necessary for energy and reproductive health. Examples of such grains are brown rice, quinoa, and oats.

Additionally, being high in fiber, whole grains can aid in balancing hormone levels and enhance reproductive health in general.

Women who are trying to get pregnant should attempt to eat a lot of fruits, vegetables, nuts, seeds, and healthy fats, such as avocado and olive oil, in addition to whole grains.

Certain meals can enhance reproductive health and aid in improving the quality of eggs. For women who are trying to get pregnant, leafy greens, berries, fatty fish, eggs, and whole grains are all healthy options.

These meals are abundant in essential nutrients, including folate, antioxidants, omega-3 fatty acids, protein, and complex carbohydrates, that are crucial for reproductive health.

Along with eating these meals, women who are trying to get pregnant should also maintain a healthy weight, engage in regular exercise, abstain from smoking, and limit their alcohol intake.

Women can increase their chances of getting pregnant and having a healthy baby by emphasizing a healthy diet and lifestyle.

Chapter 4

Hormone-Regulating Foods

The significance of essential nutrients and particular diets for better fertility and egg quality was covered in earlier chapters. In this chapter, we will concentrate on foods that can assist in hormone regulation, which is crucial for fertility and general reproductive health.

Hormones are essential to the process of reproduction. Hormone imbalances can affect fertility, menstrual periods, and ovulation. However, some meals can enhance reproductive health and help control hormone levels.

Cruciferous Plants

Indole-3-carbinol (I3C), which is abundant in cruciferous vegetables including broccoli, cauliflower, and Brussels sprouts, has anti-inflammatory properties.

Estrogen regulation, which is crucial for the balance of hormones and reproductive health, can be aided by I3C.

Additionally, studies have demonstrated a decreased risk of estrogen-dependent cancers in women who consume more cruciferous vegetables, including breast and ovarian cancer.

Flaxseeds

Lignans, which are substances that can aid in regulating hormone levels, are abundant in flaxseeds. The entire health of the reproductive system depends on the ability of lignans to minimize inflammation in the body.

In addition to lignans, omega-3 fatty acids, which we covered in Chapter 3, are also abundant in flaxseeds. Omega-3 fatty acids can enhance general reproductive health by regulating hormone synthesis.

Soy-based goods

Tofu and soy milk are two soy products that are particularly high in phytoestrogens, which are plant-based substances that can assist in regulating hormone levels.

In the body, phytoestrogens can mimic the actions of estrogen, balancing hormone levels and promoting reproductive health.

It is crucial to remember that excessive soy consumption might have a detrimental impact on hormone levels and fertility.

Moderate soy product consumption and the avoidance of highly processed soy products are recommended for women who are attempting to get pregnant.

Turmeric

Turmeric has been employed in traditional medicines since ancient times. It contains a lot of curcumin, a substance with anti-inflammatory qualities and the potential to control hormone levels.

According to research, curcumin has also been linked to improved insulin sensitivity, which is crucial for reproductive health.

Hormone levels can be affected by insulin resistance, which also raises the risk of difficulties during pregnancy and problems with fertility.

Berries

Berries, which we covered in Chapter 3, are crucial for controlling hormones. Berries are a strong source of vitamin C, which can assist in regulating hormone levels and enhancing fertility in addition to their antioxidant characteristics.

Women who are trying to get pregnant should also try to eat a lot of fruits, vegetables, whole grains, and healthy fats in addition to these foods.

To support general reproductive health, it's also critical to maintain a healthy weight and engage in regular exercise.

Certain foods can enhance reproductive health by regulating hormone levels. For women who are trying to get pregnant, cruciferous vegetables, flaxseeds, soy products, turmeric, and berries are all healthy options.

These foods are full of substances that can support hormone balance and lower inflammation in the body.

But it's crucial to remember that hormone regulation and reproductive health also depend on a balanced diet and a healthy lifestyle.

When trying to get pregnant, women should maintain a healthy weight, engage in regular exercise, abstain from smoking, and limit their alcohol intake.

Women can increase their chances of getting pregnant and having a healthy baby by emphasizing a healthy diet and lifestyle.

Chapter 5

Foods for a Healthy Pregnancy

The significance of nutrition and particular foods for fertility and reproductive health has been covered. We will concentrate on nutrients that are crucial for a healthy pregnancy in this chapter.

A woman's body undergoes significant changes during pregnancy, and both the mother and the unborn child need to eat properly.

The proper diet can encourage fetal development and growth, reduce pregnancy difficulties, and guarantee a safe pregnancy.

Protein

For the growth and development of the fetus, protein is a crucial nutrient. The amniotic fluid and placenta are vital for the development of new cells and tissues.

Women should attempt to eat at least 70 grams of protein per day while pregnant. Lean meats, poultry, fish, eggs, legumes, and nuts are all excellent sources of protein.

Iron

The formation of hemoglobin, which transports oxygen to the fetus, depends on iron. The need for iron rises during pregnancy, and women who do not get enough iron may develop iron-deficiency anemia.

Lean red meat, chicken, fish, beans, lentils, fortified cereals, and leafy green vegetables are all excellent sources of iron.

Additionally, it's vital to eat foods high in vitamin C, such as citrus fruits and strawberries, which can aid in boosting iron absorption.

Calcium

For the development of prenatal teeth and bones, calcium is crucial. Women who are pregnant should try to get at least 1000 mg of calcium daily.

Dairy goods like milk, cheese, and yogurt, leafy green vegetables, tofu, and fortified meals like orange juice and cereal are all excellent sources of calcium.

Vitamin B6

The neural tube, which eventually develops the baby's brain and spinal cord, needs folic acid to develop properly.

Pregnant women who get adequate folic acid can lower their risk of developing some birth abnormalities like spina bifida.

Women should try to get at least 600 mcg of folic acid daily while they are pregnant. Fortified cereals, leafy green vegetables, beans, and citrus fruits are excellent sources of folic acid.

The fatty acids omega-3

The development of the fetal brain and eyes depends on omega-3 fatty acids. They are crucial for maternal health as well since they can lower the risk of issues during pregnancy such as premature labor and preeclampsia.

Fatty fish, such as salmon and sardines, as well as flaxseeds, chia seeds, and walnuts, are excellent providers of omega-3 fatty acids. Women who are pregnant should try to get 200 to 300 milligrams of omega-3s daily.

Fluids

For the development and growth of the fetus as well as for the health of the mother, proper hydration is crucial. Women who are pregnant should try to drink at least 8 to 10 cups of liquids each day.

Water, milk, juice, and soup are all excellent sources of fluids. Caffeine should not be consumed in excess as it can raise the risk of miscarriage and poor birth weight.

Nutritional balance is crucial for a healthy pregnancy. Women who are expecting should try to eat a range of foods that are high in nutrients, such as protein, iron, calcium, folic acid, and omega-3 fatty acids. Additionally, it's critical to drink plenty of water and limit your caffeine intake.

Women can encourage fetal growth and development, avoid pregnancy difficulties, and guarantee a good pregnancy by emphasizing a balanced food and lifestyle.

To make sure they receive the right nutrition and care throughout their pregnancy, women should also consult with their healthcare professionals.

Chapter 6

Nutritional Advice for Fertility

In this chapter, we will go through specific dietary suggestions that can assist in enhancing fertility and raising the likelihood of conception.

These recommendations, which are supported by scientific evidence, can be beneficial for both men and women attempting to get pregnant.

Consume a Healthy Diet

A balanced diet is crucial for both reproductive health and overall wellness. Fruits such as vegetables, whole grains, lean meats, and healthy fats should make up a balanced diet.

Eat as many different fruits and veggies as you can, as they all contain different nutrients and antioxidants.

Cut out added sugars and processed foods

Processed meals and added sugars can increase insulin resistance and inflammation, both of which can be harmful to fertility.

Consuming processed foods, such as packaged snacks, fast food, and sugary beverages, should be kept to a minimum. Instead, pick entire foods that are high in nutrients and contain all the vitamins and minerals your body needs.

Pick healthy fats

Monounsaturated and polyunsaturated fats, which are healthy, are crucial for hormone balance and fertility. Avocados, nuts, seeds, olive oil, and fatty seafood are all excellent sources of healthful fats.

Trans fats should be avoided

Trans fats, which are present in processed foods, have been linked to insulin resistance and inflammation. Foods containing partially hydrogenated oils should be avoided, including fried items, baked products, and snack foods.

Consume Enough Protein

Because it contains the building blocks for hormones and reproductive organs, protein is crucial for fertility. Eat a range of lean meats, poultry, fish, eggs, beans, and nuts as well as other sources of protein.

Deciding on complex carbohydrates

Whole grains and starchy vegetables are examples of complex carbs that offer fiber and vital nutrients to boost fertility. Rather than simple carbs like those found in refined grains and sugary snacks, choose complex carbohydrates.

Consume More Vegetarian Foods

A plant-based diet has been found to promote fertility and increase the likelihood of pregnancy. The necessary nutrients and antioxidants included in plant-based foods such as fruits, vegetables, legumes, and whole grains boost reproductive health.

Limit your alcohol intake

Alcohol abuse can have a detrimental effect on fertility and raise the chance of miscarriage. Limiting alcohol use is crucial, especially when trying to get pregnant.

Keep hydrated

Taking in enough water is crucial for overall health and fertility. Aim to consume at least 8 to 10 cups of water each day and stay away from sugary beverages and excessive amounts of caffeine.

For fertility and reproductive health, eating a balanced diet is crucial. People can promote hormone control and enhance fertility by choosing nutrient-dense diets and avoiding processed foods and added sugars.

A plant-based diet, consuming adequate protein, selecting healthy fats, and drinking plenty of water can all improve fertility and increase the likelihood of conception. To create a customized nutrition plan that addresses particular needs and objectives, collaboration with a healthcare professional or registered dietitian is essential.

Chapter 7

Common Questions and Concerns about Diet and Fertility

We'll talk about some frequent queries and worries people might have about nutrition and fertility. Individuals can make educated judgments about their diet and reproductive health by being aware of these issues.

Can a diet increase fertility?

The answer is that nutrition can have a big impact on fertility. A balanced, nutrient-rich diet has been found to boost reproductive health, improve hormone management, and increase the likelihood of conception.

It's crucial to keep in mind, though, that nutrition is only one element that can affect fertility. Age, genetics, and underlying medical issues are some more factors that come into play.

Which Nutrients are Important for Fertility?

Folate, iron, zinc, vitamin D, and omega-3 fatty acids are some essential nutrients for fertility. These nutrients aid in the regulation of hormones, the quality of eggs, and reproductive health.

To ensure proper consumption of these crucial nutrients, it's crucial to eat a range of nutrient-dense meals.

Can certain Foods enhance the quality of Eggs?

Yes, some foods can enhance the quality of eggs. Antioxidant-rich foods, such as berries and leafy greens, can aid in the quality improvement and damage prevention of eggs.

Furthermore, diets high in omega-3 fatty acids, such as those containing fatty fish and walnuts, can also enhance the quality of eggs.

The Polycystic Ovary Syndrome (PCOS) and Diet: Can Diet Help?

Yes, diet can help with PCOS management. A low-glycemic index diet, which emphasizes ingesting complex carbs and avoiding simple sweets, has been demonstrated in research to improve insulin resistance and hormone balance in people with PCOS.

In addition, those with PCOS can benefit from hormone management by consuming good fats and avoiding trans fats.

Should I abstain from alcohol and caffeine while trying to conceive?

While there isn't conclusive proof that moderate alcohol and caffeine intake harm fertility, it is typically advised to limit both when trying to get pregnant.

While excessive alcohol use raises the chance of miscarriage, excessive coffee consumption can interfere with hormone control.

When attempting to conceive, it's crucial to identify the right amounts of caffeine and alcohol to consume in consultation with a healthcare professional.

Is taking Supplements While Trying to Get Pregnant Safe?

While taking supplements might help you get enough of certain essential minerals, it's crucial to use caution.

Some dietary supplements could interfere with some drugs or have unfavorable effects. Before beginning any new supplements, you should speak with a licensed nutritionist or healthcare professional.

Diet can have a significant impact on reproductive health and fertility. A healthy, nutrient-rich diet helps support hormone management, enhance egg quality, and boost pregnancy chances.

It's crucial to keep in mind, though, that nutrition is only one element that can affect fertility. Age, genetics, and underlying medical issues are some more factors that come into play.

Making decisions about one's food and reproductive health can be facilitated by addressing typical queries and worries about diet and fertility.

To create a customized nutrition plan that addresses particular needs and objectives, collaboration with a healthcare professional or registered dietitian is essential.

Conclusion

In conclusion, nutrition is crucial for fertility, and it's critical to comprehend how dietary choices affect reproductive health.

Important details on the essential nutrients that sustain fertility, foods that enhance egg quality, and dietary suggestions for maximizing fertility have been discussed in this book.

A balanced, nutrient-rich diet has been found to boost reproductive health, improve hormone management, and increase the likelihood of conception.

It is possible to ensure the appropriate consumption of essential nutrients for fertility by consuming a variety of nutrient-dense meals, such as fruits, vegetables, whole grains, lean protein sources, and healthy fats.

It can also help reproductive health to be aware of how particular diets affect hormone balance, avoid overly processed foods, and consume foods high in antioxidants and omega-3 fatty acids, for example.

It is significant to highlight that other factors besides nutrition can affect fertility. Age, genetics, and underlying medical issues are some more factors that come into play.

To create a customized nutrition plan that addresses particular needs and objectives, collaboration with a healthcare professional or registered dietitian is essential.

Even though diet has a substantial impact on fertility, it's critical to approach dietary changes from a holistic and balanced point of view.

Managing stress, getting enough sleep, exercising frequently, and abstaining from dangerous substances like excessive alcohol and tobacco use can all help reproductive health.

People can increase their chances of getting pregnant and having a healthy baby by embracing healthy eating habits and lifestyle choices.

This book's contents can be used as a guide for comprehending the connection between diet and fertility and for selecting dietary practices.

Finally, maximizing conception via nutrition necessitates a combination of knowing the essential nutrients that support reproductive health, eating a balanced and nutrient-dense diet, and attending to other factors that affect fertility.

One can increase their chances of conception and support a healthy pregnancy by approaching reproductive health holistically.

9 798391 324997